Weight loss 40+ essential tips

Weight loss 40+ essential tips

Unlocking the Fountain of Youth: 40+ Essential Tips for Effortless Weight Loss and Vibrant Health"

Shana C. Clark

Weight loss 40+ essential tips

Copyright & Disclaimer

The information provided in this book is for general informational purposes only. While every effort has been made to ensure the

Weight loss 40+ essential tips

Introduction

Weight loss awareness

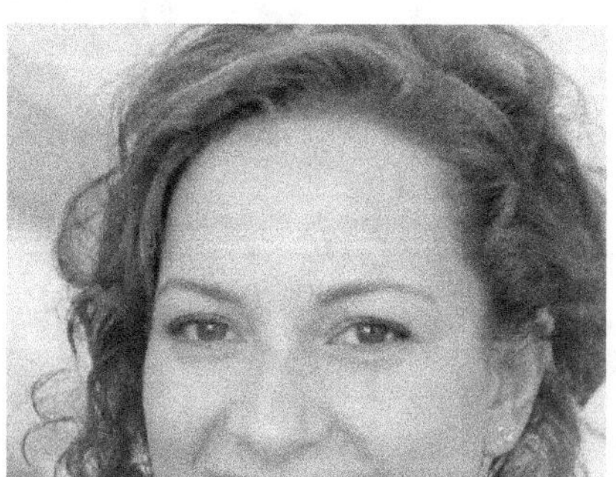

With regards to weight reduction,

there is no lack in craze diets or speedy weight loss plans. We as a whole need to feel better about the manner in which we look, yet the easy route eats less carbs, limits your nourishing admission and bombs over the long haul. Being sound isn't just about losing overabundant pounds, however adjusting the quantity of calories you consume with the quantity of calories your body utilizes, notwithstanding, suitable activity. Keeping a sound weight gets from a way of life change that requires discipline and persistence.

The initial step to a sound way of life is assuming command. You want to evaluate your weight and decide if your ongoing weight is sound, this is not set in stone by computing your Weight Record (BMI). Your BMI is determined by finding your weight and level in a BMI File Diagram. The diagram has four names for scopes of weight, "underweight", "ordinary", "overweight", and "hefty". At a singular level, BMI can be utilized as a screening device yet isn't symptomatic of the body bloatedness or wellbeing of a person. A prepared medical services supplier ought to perform fitting wellbeing appraisals to assess a singular's wellbeing status and dangers.

When you decide your BMI, you know whether you really want to free or put on weight and what that weight resembles for you. Solid weight reduction is achieved through slow and consistent weight reduction, around a couple of pounds each week. To get thinner and keep it off long haul, you should utilize a bigger number of calories than you take in and perform approximately 60 - an hour and a half of active work of moderate force four to five days per week.

Forestalling weight gain requires preparation and is a proactive method for keeping an ongoing sound weight or forestalling further weight gain. Putting together week after week feasts that authorize smart dieting propensities and integrating active work consistently, will assist you with keeping away from weight gain. By keeping away from weight gain, you can stay away from higher dangers of numerous persistent sicknesses. A few high gamble infections incorporate coronary illness, stroke, type 2 diabetes, hypertension, osteoarthritis, and a few types of disease.

You might realize a friend or family member who is battling with weight gain or you personally are having issues. Assume command and get your BMI assessed as well as biometric screening performed by your nearby Piedmont Pressing Consideration Doctor or essential consideration specialist. When you have a pattern evaluation of your ongoing wellbeing, you can start to fabricate and carry out a solid way of life that is best for you.

Weight loss 40+ essential tips

chapter 1

Find the astonishing connection between quality rest and viable weight reduction

Rest and Corpulence

In kids and youths, the connection between not getting sufficient rest and an expanded gamble of weight is deep rooted, albeit the justification for this connection is as yet being discussed. Deficient rest in youngsters can prompt metabolic abnormalities as examined before, skipping breakfast in the mornings, and expanded admission of sweet, pungent, greasy, and boring food sources.

In grown-ups, the examination is less clear. While an enormous investigation of past examinations recommends that individuals getting under 6 hours of rest around evening time are bound to be analyzed as corpulent

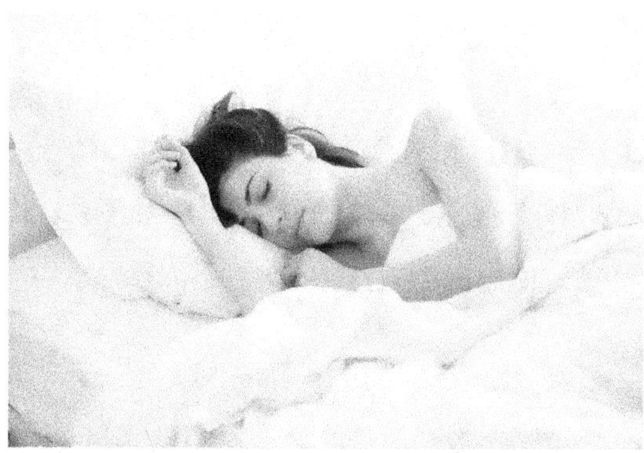

, it's provoking for these investigations to decide circumstances and logical results. Weight itself can build the gamble of creating conditions that slow down rest, similar to rest apnea and misery. It's not satisfactory in the event that getting less rest is the reason for heftiness in these examinations, on the off chance that stoutness is making the members get less rest, or maybe a blend of both. Despite the fact that more examinations are expected to comprehend this association, specialists energize further developing rest quality while treating heftiness in grown-ups.

Rest During Weight reduction
Getting sufficient, quality rest is a significant piece of a sound weight reduction plan. Above all, research has shown that terrible rest while abstaining from excessive food intake can lessen how much weight lost and energize indulging

.

Tips for Quality Rest During Weight reduction
There are numerous ways of further developing rest. The following are a couple of exploration based ways to rest better while you're attempting to get more fit:

Keep a customary rest plan: Huge swings in your rest plan or attempting to make up for lost time with rest following seven days of late evenings can cause changes in digestion and diminish insulin responsiveness

, making it simpler for glucose to be raised.

Rest in a dull room: Openness to fake light while dozing, like a television or bedside light, is related with an expanded gamble of weight gain and heftiness.

Try not to eat just before bed: Eating late may lessen the progress of weight reduction endeavors

Diminish Pressure: Constant pressure might prompt unfortunate rest and weight gain in more than one way, incorporating eating to adapt to gloomy feelings

Be a Morning person: Individuals with late sleep times might consume more calories and be at a higher gamble for weight gain

. Morning people might be bound to keep up with weight reduction when contrasted with evening people .

Weight loss 40+ essential tips

Chapter 2

Protein Ability Energizing Your Change

Proteins add to the course of energy creation by communicating and moving energy inside the cell . They can hop from one site to another, covering enormous

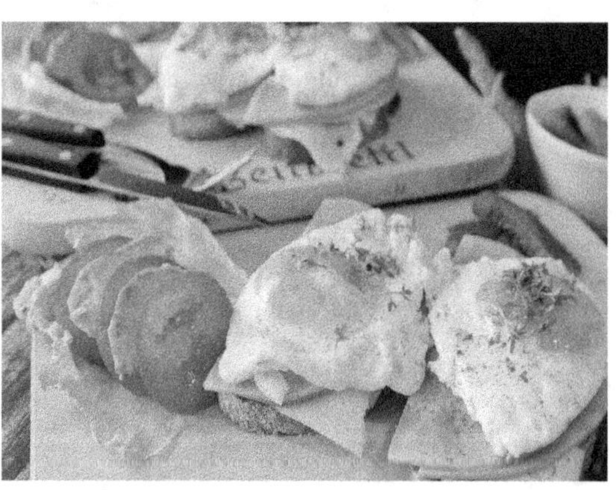

distances, and target explicit areas inside the protein . This energy move is worked with by the development of restricted methods of nonlinear beginning at the objective website, which go about as productive energy-amassing focuses . The excitation energies that yield the most elevated productivity are inside the scope of naturally important energies . Chemicals, which are proteins, assume a significant part in energy creation by catalyzing explicit responses and lessening the energy expected for reactants to arrive at their change state . Catalyst movement is directed through different components, including cutthroat and noncompetitive hindrance, allosteric guideline, and covalent change . Metabolic pathways, managed at different levels, produce energy through compound transformations and store energy as glycogen and triacylglycerol . In general, proteins and compounds assume fundamental parts in energy creation and guideline inside living creatures .

Heart and stomach tissues were gathered for metabolite profiling. Each kind of feeling brought about an alternate metabolite piece in the rodent heart and stomach tissues. In the heart tissues, EA at ST36 impacted a more extensive scope of metabolite pathways than did EA at PC6, though comparative quantities of metabolites in the stomach tissues were impacted by EA at ST36 and PC6. The pathways impacted by EA at ST36 contrasted from those impacted by EA at PC6, and a gathering of normal metabolites were contrarily directed by these two acupoints. This study showed point explicitness really regulated digestion in rodent heart and stomach tissues. The outcomes demonstrate that heart excitement might be associated with the stomach through the pericardium meridian (as depicted in customary Chinese medication), making sense of why needle therapy applied to the stomach meridian can be an elective treatment for gastric and heart sicknesses.

As a general rule, protein prerequisites fill two needs. One is as a reason for a solution (i.e., exhortation on safe eating regimens through suggesting proper dietary admissions). Variation infers a low - yet challenging to characterize - MPR. For sure, since regular weight control plans, giving adequate energy and different supplements, for the most part give extensively more than the insignificant measure of protein, the size of the MPR becomes somewhat an issue of logical interest as it were. Definition of strategy according to prescriptive issues will definitely and accurately be generally worried about fulfilling the upper scope of requests for protein and, where there is vulnerability, incorporate positive safety buffers. For this situation, it is seemingly indiscreet to take on a versatile model and diminish the MPR, regardless of whether arrangement could be arrived at on the probable lower cutoff of variation. For sure, a versatile model doesn't suggest that protein is an irrelevant supplement for the support of human wellbeing and prosperity, yet rather that pointers other than balance (N, protein, or amino corrosive) should be distinguished. In this way, the most significant measure is an ideal necessity permitting equilibrium and supporting both ideal body capability and least gamble of constant illness as displayed in Figure 1. There is expanding exploratory proof for the expected advantage of protein admissions significantly higher than the ebb and flow MPR for bone wellbeing in the old and epidemiological proof for benefit as for hypertension and ischemic coronary illness. Be that as it may, such impacts are problematic, with no conceivable system distinguished in the last option cases. Regardless, there are no quantifiable markers. This outcomes in a quandary for those endeavoring to approach prescriptive dietary rules. According to this viewpoint, it is presumably insightful to hold current qualities as a functional catalyst (basically those that are protected) until it becomes conceivable to measure the advantages (and any dangers) of protein admissions inside the versatile reach.

The other reason for prerequisite suggestions is as a demonstrative sign of deficiency risk, frequently inside an epidemiological setting in which populace bunches as opposed to people are thought of. For this situation, markers used to appraise predominance of infection states or shortage risk are painstakingly picked to figure out some kind of harmony between misleading up-sides and bogus negatives. The fundamental ramifications of variation for assessing hazard of lack as admissions tumble to not as much as necessity levels is an emotional decrease in the commonness of chance for most populaces contrasted with that surveyed concurring with the conventional model, which doesn't represent transformation. This happens in light of the fact that the necessity and admission can be thought to be connected and in light of the fact that the genuine MPR and safe admission determined from it will be lower. As in the prescriptive setting, this generally safe of lack applies just to that of being not able to keep up with NB after full variation with in any case healthfully sufficient weight control plans fulfilling the energy requests. Healthfully sufficient eating regimens containing protein admissions at such low levels are probably going to be extremely uncommon, and whether such populaces appreciate ideal protein-related wellbeing concerning safe capability, bone wellbeing, or some other capability is a different issue and should be tended to in that capacity. According to this point of view, it follows that upkeep of NB can presently not be utilized as a proxy of sufficient protein-related wellbeing and that ongoing absence of quantifiable elective markers is not a good reason for overlooking the issue of variation.

Chapter 3

Calories Divulged

How much energy in food or drink is estimated in calories.

Why are calories significant?

You really want energy from calories for your body to appropriately work. Your body utilizes this energy to appropriately work. To remain at around similar weight, the calories your body uses ought to be equivalent to how much calories you eat and drink.

In the event that you don't involve similar measure of calories as you eat and drink, your body weight might change. For instance:

you're probably going to gain weight in the event that you eat and drink a greater number of calories than you use. This is on the grounds that your body stores the additional energy as fat you're probably going to get more fit assuming you eat and drink less calories than you use. This is on the grounds that your body involves its put away fat for energy

- Day to day calories

Calorie data is much of the time given in kcals, which is short for kilocalories. It might likewise be given in kJ, which is short for kilojoules.

As an aide:

a typical man needs 2,500kcal per day

a typical lady needs 2,000kcal per day

This could be different in view of your:

age

weight

level

how much activity you do

The 20 food that contain 'zero' calories:

1. Apples

2. Apricots

3. Beetroot

4. Broccoli

5. Cauliflower

6. Celery

7. Watercress

8. Cucumber

9. Garlic

10. Grapefruit

11. Green beans

12. Kale

13. Leeks

14. Lemons

15. Lettuce

16. Onions

17. Raspberries

18. Strawberries

19. Swede

20. Watermelon

Weight loss 40+ essential tips

Chapter 4

an urgent step towards a better you

15 ways to work on yourself every day

Prepare. Likewise with numerous things, personal growth ought to begin with an arrangement. Plan what you need to accomplish in the following couple of days, weeks, or months. Record plans for the day so you don't sit around idly recollecting what you really want to finish. Keeping a journal or diary can likewise assist you with seeing what you got along admirably and what you could improve.

Put forth objectives. Make present moment and long haul objectives for yourself, and set time restricts so you can keep tabs on your development. The more you're ready to imagine where you need to go, the more inspiration you'll need to keep arriving at that objective.

Acknowledge demands. Escaping your usual range of familiarity can assist you with acknowledging potential you never at any point realized you had. Try not to avoid something since it alarms you (for however long it's not unlawful or hazardous, obviously). It's smarter to fizzle and develop from your slip-ups than to never attempt.

Gain some new useful knowledge. Whether it's another dialect, music, cooking, or a game, mastering another expertise can assist you with extending your sweet spot and give you certainty to attempt all the more new things.

Quit griping. Releasing pressure every so often can be solid. Be that as it may, griping can here and there get you stalled by regrettable contemplations. Attempt to zero in on the positive, and don't flounder in errors or difficulties.

Practice care. Getting soiled down in the pressure and hustle of day to day existence is simple. Have a go at taking a couple of seconds during your day to think, which can assist you with easing pressure and practice care.

Enjoy a hearty chuckle. Regardless of how occupied you get, remember to have a good time. Chuckling is helpful. Invest energy with loved ones who make you snicker or watch your #1 satire show.

Limit your screen time. These days, it's very simple to go down the dark hole of virtual entertainment, PC games, and television. A lot of time spent taking a gander at your screen can be harming to your wellbeing and remove time from other more useful exercises.

Figure out how to say no. Really extraordinary to express yes to new encounters, you likewise need to figure out how to say no. Try not to genuinely regret safeguarding your own prosperity when you're overpowered, exhausted, or overtired. Burnout can hurt your wellbeing and inward feeling of harmony.

accomplished more than others. Attempt to utilize your opportunity to the fullest by getting up ahead of schedule or cutting out chance to work out. Not in the least does getting your body going assist you with remaining genuinely solid, however it additionally assists you with keeping on track, positive, and stimulated.

Get sufficient rest. Getting 7-8 hours of value rest every night is fundamental, so don't hold back on your rest. Permit yourself to loosen up, unwind, and get sufficient rest so that you're prepared for the following day.

Hydrate. Remaining hydrated is fundamental to keeping up with your weight, state of mind, and wellbeing. Ensure you are drinking water over the course of the day and skirt the sweet beverages and soft drinks.

Water and Fiber Sorcery

Air, Water and Fiber - secret elements for leanness

Iam cutting. Do you have any idea about what this implies? It implies yearning, hostility and endless desires… essentially for a great many people, yet not really for me. At the point when I'm on a weight reduction diet I'm rarely eager…

well never, except if I screw up my feast timing, since I'm too in the middle of doing science

Do you think about how I oversee it not to be eager in calorie deficiency? - Everything without a doubt revolves around the right food decisions. I understand what you think now, we heard it multiple times; eat veggies, don't eat low quality food, decrease sugar and the wide range of various blablabla…

Presently hang on for a couple of moments and consider it. What do the vast majority of the standard proposals share practically speaking? There are two significant things: decrease calories and increment food volume.

There are 3 'enchantment' food parts that can do both - air, water and fiber (and you can get them for (nearly) free! you don't have to pay loads of cash for extravagant, futile fat killers). Air and water have zero calories. Fiber has a couple, nonetheless, significantly less than different supplements, as it isn't separated by our bodies. Our stomach microbes use fiber as energy supply and convert the extras into short chain unsaturated fats that are taken up by our bodies to help numerous significant cycles; expanded satiety is one of them. Fiber is perfect!

- Promotion

Consequently, sinewy vegetables and low-sugar natural products are extraordinary food decisions when you need to shed pounds. Obviously, you definitely realize that foods grown from the ground are great for wellbeing and weight reduction.

What I need to show you are a few offbeat food sources that diminish craving and assist you with making your weight reduction diet more manageable.

I love fat-diminished coconut flour! It has 40 g fiber for every 100 g! That is a great deal, hence it is super satisfying. The leftover macros aren't really awful either, around 20 g of each, carbs, protein and fat.

Be that as it may, you can't have everything. Planning food with coconut flour is a piece interesting, due to its high fiber content and its pastiness. My answer for this issue is thickener (have I previously referenced that I love it?). Whenever I use coconut flour for my recipes, I join it with thickener, which gives a more tacky or velvety surface.

- Look at what I use coconut flour for:

Breakfast bowl - Super satisfying, heavenly and has pretty respectable macros: 283 kcal/15 g carbs/32 g protein/10 g fat/18 g fiber

Recipe: Blend 33 g coconut flour, 33 g white hemp protein, 1/3 cup unsweetened almond milk, 1/4 tsp. thickener and 1 serving vanilla FlavDrops (from myprotein) and top with 100 g strawberries (<-low-sugar natural products, loads of water, fiber and not an excessive number of calories *hint*)

Speedy bars - astounding as a fast feast and an extraordinary choice for voyaging (you would rather not eat all the poo you ordinarily get on the way, truly). You could dice the bars and use them as breakfast grain substitution (remember to finish off with strawberries, strawberries are perfect!

Approx. wholesome data: 267 kcal/10 g carbs/33 g protein/10 g fat/15 g

Recipe:

Fixings: 300 g white hemp protein (you can utilize green hemp in the event that you add more cacao powder), 250 g coconut ridicule (fat reduced), 25 g cacao powder, 10 g xanthan gum, a touch of salt, no-calorie sugar (discretionary, however suggested) and 650-750 ml fluid

Bearings: 1. Blend all dry ingredients 2. Add water gradually why blending the combination in with a hand mixer 3. Work the blend with you hands until it gets a tacky ish surface 4. Partition in 8 equivalent segments 5. Pack and wrap the bars: Put some stick foil into an estimating cup, put in one blend segment, press solidly, take it out (simply pull up the grip film) and close the grip film

Alright, got it. It's not excessively difficult to expand fiber and water content of my eating routine. Yet, how in the world do I get air into my food?

Likewise for this I have an answer: my zero calorie cushion. As I previously referenced above, thickener is perfect! It is perfect for richness, tenacity and for making air in water emulsions (have I at any point referenced that my PhD was on making emulsions Thickener permits you to make air bubbles that are encircled by water = cushion. What you eat is essentially air and water! What you really want presently is adding flavor to your zero calorie cushion (eating simply air and water is some way or another wearing as I would like to think out). This is the way my dearest zero calorie espresso cushion was conceived!

You will find the point by point emulsification convention in my new recipe book. - > Coming out extremely, soon! To keep awake to information, buy into my email list (in the event that you haven't yet).

Chapter 5

Advantages of Active work

For beforehand stationary people, a sluggish movement in active work has been suggested with the goal that 30 minutes of work-out everyday is

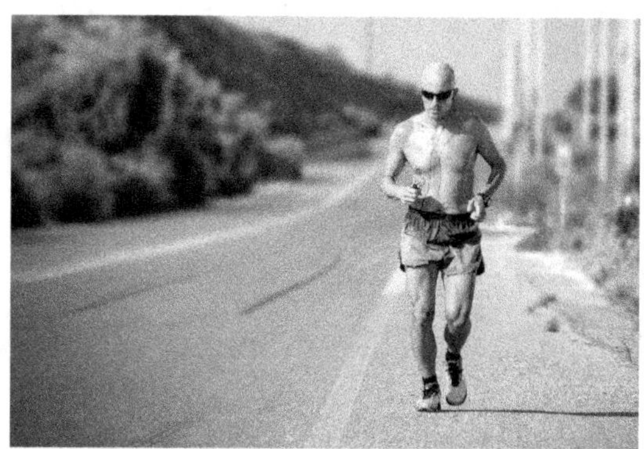

accomplished following half a month of steady development. This may likewise apply to some tactical faculty, particularly newcomers or reservists reviewed to deployment ready who might be entering administration from already exceptionally stationary ways of life. The action objective has been communicated as an expansion in energy use of 1,000 kcal/wk

(Jakicic et al., 1999; Pate et al., 1995), albeit this amount might be lacking to forestall weight recover. For that reason, a week by week objective of 2,000 to 3,000 kcal of added action might be vital (Klem et al., 1997; Schoeller et al., 1997). Hence, mental groundwork for how much action important to keep up with weight reduction should start while shedding pounds (Brownell, 1999).

For some people, changing movement levels is seen as more terrible than making progress with dietary propensities. Separating a 30-minute day to day work out "remedy" into 10-minute sessions has been displayed to increment consistence over that of longer sessions (Jakicic et al., 1995, Pate et al., 1995). In any case, north of a 18-month time span, people who performed short episodes of actual work didn't encounter upgrades in long haul weight reduction, cardiorespiratory wellness, or actual work cooperation in examination with the people who performed longer episodes of activity. Some proof recommends that home gym equipment (e.g., a treadmill) improves the probability of customary activity and is related with more prominent long haul weight reduction (Jakicic et al., 1999). Also, individual inclinations are central contemplations in decisions of movement.

While strength preparing or opposition practice is joined with oxygen consuming action, long haul results might be preferable over those with heart stimulating exercise alone (Poirier and Despres, 2001; Sothern et al., 1999). Since strength preparing will in general form muscle, loss of fit weight might be limited and the overall loss of muscle to fat ratio might be expanded. An additional advantage is the lessening of the diminishing in resting metabolic rate related with weight reduction, perhaps as an outcome of saving or upgrading lean weight.

However important as exercise seems to be, the current examination writing on overweight people demonstrates that exercise programs alone don't create critical weight reduction in the populaces contemplated. It ought to be underlined, in any case, that countless such examinations have been led with moderately aged Caucasian ladies driving stationary ways of life. The disappointment of activity alone to deliver critical weight reduction might be on the grounds that the neurochemical components that direct eating conduct make people make up for the calories consumed in practice by expanding food (calorie) consumption. While practice projects can bring about a normal weight reduction of 2 to 3 kg temporarily (Blair, 1993; Pavlou et al., 1989a; Skender et al., 1996; Wadden and Sarwer, 1999), result improves fundamentally when active work is joined with dietary mediation. For instance, when actual work was joined with a decreased calorie diet and way of life change, a weight reduction of 7.2 kg was accomplished following a half year to 3 years of follow-up (Blair, 1993). Actual work in addition to eat less carbs creates improved results than one or the other eating regimen or active work alone (Blair, 1993; Dyer, 1994; Pavlou et al., 1989a, 1989b; Perri et al., 1993). What's more, weight recapture is fundamentally more uncertain when actual work is joined with some other weight-decrease routine (Blair, 1993; Klem et al., 1997). Proceeded trail behind weight reduction is related with further developed result in the event that the action plan is observed and adjusted as a component of this development (Kayman et al., 1990).

While studies have shown that tactical volunteers had the option to lose huge measures of weight during introductory section preparing through practice alone, the confined time accessible to consume dinners during preparing most likely added to this weight reduction (Lee et al., 1994).

Conduct AND Way of life Alteration

The utilization of conduct and way of life alteration in weight the executives depends on a collection of proof that individuals become or stay overweight as the consequence of modifiable propensities or ways of behaving and that by changing those ways of behaving, weight can be lost and the misfortune can be kept up with. The essential objectives of social procedures for weight control are to increment active work and to diminish caloric admission by changing dietary patterns (Brownell and Kramer, 1994; Wilson, 1995). A subcategory of change in behavior patterns, ecological administration, is examined in the following segment. Social treatment, which was presented during the 1960s, might be given to a solitary individual or to gatherings of clients. Normally, people partake in 12 to 20 week after week meetings that last from 1 to 2 hours each (Brownell and

Kramer, 1994), with an objective of weight reduction in the scope of 1 to 2 lb/wk (Brownell and Kramer, 1994). Previously, social methodologies were applied as independent medicines to just alter dietary patterns and diminish caloric admission. Notwithstanding, more as of late, these therapies have been utilized in blend with low-calorie eats less carbs, clinical nourishment treatment, sustenance training, practice programs, checking, pharmacological specialists, and social help to advance weight reduction, and as a part of upkeep programs.

Self-Checking and Criticism

Self-checking of dietary admission and active work, which empowers the person to foster a feeling of responsibility, is one of the foundations of conduct treatment. Patients are approached to keep a day to day food journal in which they record what and the amount they have eaten, when and where the food was devoured, and the setting wherein the food was devoured (e.g., what else they were doing at that point, what they were feeling, and who else was there). Moreover, patients might be approached to track their everyday proactive tasks. Self-checking of food admission is frequently connected with a somewhat quick decrease in food consumption and subsequent weight reduction (Blundell, 2000; Goris et al., 2000). This decrease in food admission is accepted to result from expanded attention to food consumption as well as worry about what the dietitian or sustenance advisor will think about the patient's eating conduct. The data acquired from the food journals likewise is utilized to recognize individual and ecological elements that add to gorging and to choose and carry out suitable weight reduction procedures for the individual (Wilson, 1995). The equivalent might be valid for active work observing, albeit little examination has been led around here. Self-checking likewise gives a way to specialists and patients to assess which methods are working and the way that adjustments of eating conduct or movement are adding to weight reduction. Late work has recommended that customary self-observing of body weight is a valuable assistant to change in conduct programs (Jeffery and French, 1999).

Weight loss 40+ essential tips

Conclusion

Nourishment Instruction

The board of overweight and corpulence requires the dynamic cooperation of the person. Nourishment experts can give people a base of data that permits them to settle on proficient food decisions.

Nourishment instruction is particular from sustenance directing, albeit the items cross-over impressively. Nourishment advising and dietary administration will generally zero in more straightforwardly on the persuasive, close to home, and mental issues related with the ongoing undertaking of weight reduction and weight the executives. It tends to the how of conduct changes in the dietary field. Sustenance training then again, gives essential data about the logical underpinning of nourishment that empowers individuals to arrive at informed conclusions about food, cooking strategies, eating out, and assessing segment sizes. Sustenance training programs additionally may give data on the job of nourishment in wellbeing advancement and sickness counteraction, sports nourishment, and sustenance for pregnant and lactating ladies. Compelling sustenance schooling grants nourishment information and its utilization in solid living. For instance, it makes sense of the idea of energy balance in weight the executives in an available, pragmatic way that has importance to the singular's way of life, remembering that for the tactical setting.

Composed materials arranged by different government offices or by charitable wellbeing associations can be utilized successfully to give nourishment schooling. Be that as it may, composed materials are best when used to support casual homeroom or directing meetings and to give explicit data, for example, a table of the calorie content of food sources. The arrangement of instruction programs changes significantly, and can incorporate conventional classes, casual gathering gatherings, or video chatting. A typical foundation among bunch individuals is useful (yet rare conceivable).

Instructive arrangements that give commonsense and applicable sustenance data for program members are the best. For instance, some tactical weight-the board programs incorporate field outings to post trades, eateries (inexpensive food and others), motion pictures, and different spots where food is bought or devoured (Vorachek, 1999).

The contribution of life partners and other relatives in a training program improves the probability that different individuals from the family will roll out long-lasting improvements, which thusly upgrades the probability that the program members will keep on getting in shape or keep up with weight reduction (Hart et al., 1990; Hertzler and Schulman, 1983; Sperry, 1985). Specific consideration should be coordinated to association of those in the family who are probably going to search for and plan food. Except if the program member lives alone, nourishment the executives is seldom viable without the inclusion of relatives.

www.ingramcontent.com/pod-product-compliance
Lightning Source LLC
Chambersburg PA
CBHW070726260726
48660CB00007B/2744